The Better Bath vol. 1: Bath Bomb Recipes for Better Health

Written by Lacey Jones

Disclaimer:

The information contained in this book is for general information purposes only.

While we endeavor to keep the information up to date and correct, we make no representations or warranties of any kind, express or implied, about the completeness, accuracy, reliability, suitability or availability with respect to the book or the information, products, services, or related graphics contained in the book for any purpose. Any reliance you place on such information is therefore strictly at your own risk.

None of the information in this this book is meant to be construed as medical advice. Essential oils are powerful compounds. Consult with a medical professional prior to making changes that could impact your health.

Contents

Chapter 1: The Bath Bomb

Most people have no clue what to expect the first time they drop a bath bomb into the tub. The compact little ball they were holding in their hand moments earlier explodes into a flurry of bubbles and colors, releasing the oils and butters contained inside into the tub. As the essential oils in the bath bomb are released, the fragrance of the oils slowly fills the room, creating an environment that's relaxing and soothing.

While bath bombs might seem a little strange at a glance, the reaction that causes the bubbling is actually caused by adding water to two relatively harmless ingredients. The two ingredients that cause the reaction are *baking soda*, an item most people already have in their home, and *citric acid*, which can be purchased at most supermarkets or online. Combine baking soda and citric acid and add water and you get a reaction that produces carbon dioxide. When you toss a bath bomb in the tub, the little bubbles you see are the carbon dioxide bubbles that are escaping the bath bomb.

Sounds pretty simple, right?

Well, it's slightly more complicated than that, but once you get the hang of it, you'll be making all sorts of fragrant and therapeutic bath bombs in no time at all. You can make them in all sizes and the shapes you make them in are only limited by your ability to find items that can be used as molds.

Tossing a bath bomb in the tub and letting the tiny bubbles massage you as it goes off and fills the room with fragrance is a great way to relax and unwind. A number of compounds like butters, vegetable oils and essential oils can be added to bath bombs to add therapeutic value. Choose the right ingredients and they'll leave your skin feeling soft and supple, and you'll get out of the tub feeling happy and healthy.

Once you're done reading this book, you'll be able to make completely natural bath bombs that are full of ingredients that are good for you at a fraction of the cost of what they'd cost if you bought them from the store. You'll be able to use them whenever you'd like, and they can be given as gifts that all the ladies in your life will love. I've yet to find someone who didn't appreciate a good bath bomb!

This book is intended to be a quick and easy guide for anyone who's looking to get started making bath bombs. Once we've explored the basics, we'll get right into the recipes and you'll be provided step-by-step instructions for making a number of amazing bath bomb. If you're new to making bath bombs, you're going to want to read the first 5 chapters very closely. If you're a seasoned vet, you can skip ahead to chapter 6 if you'd like and go straight to the recipes.

Chapter 2: The Golden Rule

When it comes to measuring ingredients for your bath bombs, there's one steadfast rule you need to keep in mind. The ratio of baking soda to citric acid needs to be kept at 2-to-1. What this means is no matter what measurement you're using, be it tablespoons, cups, ounces, or even pounds, you need to use 2 parts baking soda for every 1 part citric acid that you use.

If you're using ounces, you'll need 2 ounces of baking soda for every ounce of citric acid used. If you're using tablespoons, use 2 tablespoons baking soda and 1 tablespoon citric acid. You'll end up with a rather small bath bomb, but you get the point. This book uses cups as the measurement, and there isn't a single recipe that deviates from the 2 cups baking soda and 1 cup citric acid formula.

Remember this rule. If you don't get the ratio right, you'll end up with bath bombs that go off with a whimper instead of a bang.

Chapter 3: Gathering Ingredients and Supplies

Supplies fall into two basic categories. On one hand, you have the small handful of inexpensive supplies that are required in order to make bath bombs. On the other hand, you have all sorts of additional ingredients that can be added to enhance your bath bombs that run the gamut from being affordable to being so expensive that a small vial will set you back a car payment.

First, let's take a look at the ingredients you're going to need in your bath bombs:

- **Baking soda.**
- **Citric acid.**
- **Corn starch.**
- **Epsom salt.**
- **Water or witch hazel.**
- **Some sort of vegetable oil.**

Those are the only ingredients that are required, and even the corn starch can be left out if you don't mind your bath bombs sinking to the bottom of the tub.

Making a bath bomb using just the ingredients above will result in a functional bath bomb that fizzes and releases vegetable oil and Epsom salt into the tub, but does little else. This bath bomb will condition and moisturize the skin, and it may have other properties depending on the type of vegetable oil used, but it won't be anything special. There won't be any colors or fragrances released, and the end result is a bath bomb that might be fun to watch the first time you set it off, but really isn't anything to write home about.

That's where the optional ingredients come into play. The following ingredients can be added to bath bombs to enhance them from both an aesthetic and a therapeutic standpoint:

- **Designer salts.**
- **Dried herbs and flower petals.**
- **Essential oils.**
- **Glitter.**
- **Plant butters.**
- **Small candies and sugars.**

Some bath bomb experts also recommend adding a small amount of *Sodium Lauryl Sulfate (SLS)* to bath bomb recipes to get them to bubble and foam as much as the commercial bath bombs do. I don't use this ingredient in my bath bombs because it's added to give the *illusion* of a more effective bath bomb, but doesn't contribute anything other than a little more frothing action. It's a synthetic chemical, and I like to keep my bath as natural as possible.

As far as supplies go, you're going to need a handful of items on hand. You're going to need a pair of glass bowls and a whisk for mixing ingredients. You're also going to want a spray bottle that can be used to mist water or witch hazel onto the bath bomb mix and a small saucepan you can use to gently melt the oils and butters if it's cold and they're in a solid state.

The last item you're going to need is a mold into which the bath bombs can be pressed. All sorts of items can be used as molds, with silicon and plastic molds being the most popular. Bath bomb molds that are designed specifically for bath bombs are available, but you aren't limited to using just that type of mold. Look for candy molds, Christmas ornaments that can be taken apart, and anything else that's made from a non-reactive material that can be used as a mold. I've even seen cookie cutters used as molds to good effect.

Baking Soda and Citric Acid

We already touched upon these ingredients briefly in Chapter 2, but let's take a closer look at both of them.

Baking soda, also known as *bicarbonate of soda*, is an item most people already have in their home. It's found in most stores that sell baking supplies and can also be purchased at department stores, health food stores and pharmacies. Failing that, you can order it online, and a big box will only set you back a couple bucks. If you're planning on making a lot of bath bombs, you can get a 4-pound box of Arm and Hammer baking soda from Amazon.com for less than $10.

Don't confuse baking soda with baking powder when it comes to your bath bomb recipes. Baking powder contains baking soda, but it also has a couple additional ingredients that aren't needed as far as bath bombs go.

Citric acid might prove marginally more difficult to find in the store. Most supermarkets carry it in their baking supplies section, but it isn't as common an item as baking soda. If your local grocer doesn't carry it, try checking the cleaning supplies section of your local department store. Pharmacies may also carry it in the skin care section. If you don't feel like hunting it down locally, it can be ordered online for less than $5 per pound.

Don't forget the Bath Bomb Golden Rule. Use 2 parts baking soda to 1 part citric acid in your recipes to ensure your bath bomb works correctly.

Corn Starch

Corn starch is a powdered starch that's made from grains of corn. It's created by grinding the dried endosperm of the corn grains into a fine powder. If you cook a lot, you might already have corn starch in the pantry since it's used to thicken gravies and sauces, and it's used in a number of baked goods. When added to bath bombs, corn starch is there to act as a bulking and binding agent. It adds volume to the bath bombs, helps them stick together and ensures they float on the surface of the water while they do their thing.

The amount of corn starch used depends on whether Epsom salt and other dry ingredients are added. If no dry ingredients other than baking soda and citric acid are used, corn starch is used in an amount equal to half the citric acid. If Epsom salt or other dry ingredients are used, the amount of corn starch added to the recipe is usually reduced.

You can buy cornstarch at your local grocery store, or it can be ordered online. You can get it for a couple bucks per pound, unless you want to go organic. Then expect to pay at least $5 per pound.

Epsom Salt (and Sea Salts)

Epsom salt is a key ingredient in the bath bomb recipes in this book. While it's called a salt, Epsom salt is actually a mineral compound made up of magnesium and sulfate. It's added to add volume to the bath bombs and carries a number of benefits with it. Epsom salt is a natural remedy for a variety of ailments and has long been used in health and beauty applications.

The magnesium found in Epsom salt is readily absorbed into the skin. It plays a number of roles in the body, including reducing inflammation and improving nerve and muscle functions. The sulfates found in Epsom salt help flush out toxins. A soak in a tub with Epsom salt dissolved in it can help you relax and may soothe any aches and pains you've been suffering from. When Epsom salt is added to bath bombs, it's usually added at a quarter of the amount of citric acid. For example, if one cup of citric acid is used, ¼ cup of Epsom salt would be added.

Epsom salt can be purchased at your local pharmacy or drug store. You can also get it online for $2 to $3 per pound.

Other designer sea salts like Himalayan pink sea salt can also be added to bath bombs. These sea salts are usually added to add an interesting look to the bath bomb, but will also add nutrients and minerals to the bath. These sea salts can be purchased in health food stores and boutiques that cater to people who make their own cosmetics and bath products. They can also be ordered online, if you don't feel like hunting them down.

Water or Witch hazel

Water or witch hazel can be used interchangeably in bath bombs. It's added as the final step before packing the bath bomb into the mold in order to get it damp enough to where it can be molded. The easiest way to add it to the bath bomb mix is to put it in a spray bottle and spray a fine mist onto the mix. A light misting is less likely to set off the reaction between the baking soda and citric acid.

I prefer witch hazel over water because it foams less and adds a handful of benefits to the bath bomb.

Witch hazel is an astringent liquid produced from the witch hazel plant, a shrub that's native to Canada and North America. Historically, it has seen use as a medicine used by Native Americans and can be used for blemish control, to soothe and heal stubborn rashes and to reduce inflammation. Witch hazel can be purchased from most drug stores and pharmacies, or you can get it online. 12 ounces will cost you less than $10 bucks and can be used to create multiple batches of bath bombs.

There are a number of fragranced witch hazels on the market. I normally use unscented witch hazel, but lately I've been experimenting with the fragranced varieties. One of my personal favorites is the Cucumber Witch Hazel with Aloe Vera from Thayers.

Vegetable Oils

Unrefined vegetable oils, also known as *carrier oils*, are added to bath bombs because they add a number of benefits.

For one, they act as an emollient and help disperse the other ingredients into the water as the bomb melts. Without vegetable oils, most of the ingredients in the bath bomb would float to the surface of the water. Carrier oils help spread at least some of the ingredients out through the water column.

The vegetable oils that are commonly used in bath bombs are known as carrier oils because they carry the essential oils used in the recipes deep beneath the surface of the skin. Carrier oils allow the body to take full advantage of the many benefits of essential oils.

The last thing vegetable oils do is help keep the bath bomb mixture bound together after it's pressed into the molds. There's a fine line between using too much oil and not enough oil, so you have to be careful not to overdo it.

Here are some of the more common vegetable oils used in bath bombs:

- **Almond oil.**
- **Apricot kernel oil.**
- **Avocado oil.**
- **Castor oil.**
- **Coconut oil.**
- **Grapeseed oil.**
- **Olive oil.**

Most vegetable oils add moisturizing properties to the bath bombs they're added to. They can also add a handful of other benefits like creating a protective barrier on the skin and helping heal skin that's been ravaged by age. The best vegetable oils for bath bombs are ones that have a relatively mild fragrance that doesn't compete with the essential oils that are added to the mix. Go with virgin, unrefined oils instead of the refined versions of the oil whenever possible.

Plant Butters

Plant butters are butters that are made from oils that usually come from the seeds or nuts of plants. They tend to have stronger fragrances than vegetable oils, so the amount and type of plant butters you use has to be carefully considered.

They're an optional ingredient in bath bomb recipes and can be added for a number of reasons. They have moisturizing properties and can be used to help promote better skin health. Plant butters are usually a solid at room temperature, so they can also be added to bath bombs to help hold them together. You have to be careful not to rely on butters too much because they will start to melt at warmer temperatures. A bath bomb with a lot of butter in it can lose its shape and fall apart as temperatures begin to climb.

The following butters can be used in bath bombs:

- **Aloe vera butter.**
- **Apricot kernel butter.**
- **Avocado butter.**
- **Cocoa butter.**
- **Cupuacu butter.**
- **Illipe butter.**
- **Kokum butter.**
- **Mango butter.**
- **Shea butter.**

Use plant butters in small amounts for best results. A tablespoon or two of butter will go a long way. Use too much and you'll be left with bath bombs that won't harden and will go soft when the temperature rises.

Essential Oils

Of all the ingredients that are added to bath bombs, essential oils require the most attention. Essential oils are the fragrant compounds found within plants that give them their characteristic smell. When you smell a plant, leaf, tree or flower, what you actually smell is the essential oils contained within. These fragrant oils are collected and bottled up and sold under the moniker essential oils.

Essential oils are added to bath bombs for two reasons. The first reason is to add natural fragrance to the bath bombs. Essential oils typically smell like a concentrated version of the plants they came from. Lavender essential oil smells like lavender flowers, eucalyptus essential oil smells like eucalyptus trees and rose oil smells like roses, just to name a few. Essential oils can be used on their own, or they can be combined to make fragrance blends that mix and meld familiar fragrances.

Another consideration that must be made is the therapeutic properties of the essential oils being used. Essential oils can do everything from clearing up skin problems and healing damaged skin to improving your mood and leaving you feeling invigorated and ready to take on the world. While essential oils have been used to treat various illnesses and ailments for thousands of years, the scientific world is just now starting to realize just how beneficial they can be.

Essential oils are extremely powerful and are best when used in small amounts. They can interact with certain types of prescription medications, enhancing or dulling the effect of the medication, and a number of essential oils shouldn't be used by pregnant women or people who have certain health conditions, so always check with your doctor before adding new essential oils to your bath products.

You might see some recipes that call for use of fragrance oils instead of essential oils. These recipes might smell great, but they won't have the same therapeutic benefits as essential oils. The upside to using the occasional fragrance oil is you get fragrances that aren't possible when you're using essential oils alone. None of the recipes in this book call for fragrance oils. You can experiment with them on your own if you'd like.

Chapter 4: Making Your First Bath Bomb

If you're new to the world of bath bombs, pay close attention to the information in this chapter. This chapter lays out the basic bath bomb that will be used to make the most of the recipes in the book. Once you've mastered the basics, making bath bombs becomes a breeze.

Let's take a look at each of the steps required to make a bath bomb in detail.

Step 1: Combine the dry ingredients.

I prefer to do this step in two parts. First, I combine the baking soda and citric acid and make sure it's completely mixed together. This can be done by adding the baking soda and citric acid to a glass bowl and using a whisk to mix it together. It can also be done by sifting the two ingredients into the bowl, which will help ensure there aren't any solid chunks of baking soda or citric acid left after they're mixed.

It's absolutely critical that you have the baking soda and citric acid mixed thoroughly. If there are areas that aren't combined, those areas won't fizz when you toss the bath bomb in the tub.

Next, I add the rest of the dry ingredients and stir them in. This includes flower petals, tea leaves, glitter and anything else I'm adding that isn't wet. The only dry ingredients I don't stir in are ingredients I plan on using to decorate the outside of the bath bomb. It isn't as critical that these ingredients are thoroughly blended into the mix. Give them a good stir and they should be good to go.

Step 2: Combine the wet ingredients.

In this step, I combine all of the wet ingredients except for the water or witch hazel, which is added in the next step. Wet ingredients that are added in Step 2 include essential oils, butters, vegetable oils and any other wet ingredients I've decided I want to add.

If it's cold, the butters and vegetable oils could be in a solid state. They need to be gently melted over low heat until they reach liquid form. Let them cool for a bit before adding the essential oils and stirring them in, or you might damage some of the beneficial compounds in the essential oils.

Once I've got all ingredients in their liquid state, I add them to a glass bowl and whisk them together until they're thoroughly combined.

Step 3: Combine the wet and the dry ingredients.

In this step, I combine the wet and the dry ingredients. Don't just dump all of the wet ingredients into the dry ingredients because doing so can set off the reaction between the citric acid and baking soda. Add the wet ingredients to the dry ingredient (not the other way around!) slowly and stir them in.

If the mix starts to bubble while you're adding the wet ingredients, cover the area that's bubbling with dry ingredients and quickly stir it in, and the reaction should stop. I've found this step is easiest when I forget all about using mixing tools and just dive right in with my hands. Kneading the wet ingredients into the dry ingredients allows me to really work them together, and it makes breaking up any lumps that form easier than trying to hunt them down with the whisk.

Be aware that the citric acid can sting if you have open scratches, sores or scrapes on your hand. You're also going to be coming in direct contact with the essential oils, which may or may not be an issue depending on the types of oils you're using and the amount they're being used in. Nitrile gloves can be used to protect your hands.

Step 4: Get the mix to the right consistency.

While all of the steps are important, this is the most important step as far as getting your bath bombs to stay together is concerned. You have to make sure the bath bomb mix is the right consistency before it's packed into the molds, or your bath bombs are going to fall apart when you pull them out of the mold. It can be difficult to get the consistency right when you're first starting out. Once you've made a few batches, you'll be able to tell when you've got things right, but the first few batches can be hit and miss.

You want the mix to be slightly damp to the touch. When you pick up a handful of the mix and squeeze it, it should stay tightly packed when you open your hand. If it's too dry, it'll crumble. If it's too wet, it'll slump over.

This is where the spray bottle full of water or witch hazel comes into play. If the mix is too dry, I set the spray bottle to the fine mist setting and spray a couple sprays onto the mix. Next, I work the liquid into the mix and test it again by squeezing it. If it's still too dry, I'll add a couple more sprays and work them in.

Sometimes you'll find your mixture is too damp. If it's just a little bit too damp, you can usually add more citric acid and baking soda to get it to the right consistency. Remember to keep it blended at a 2-to-1 ration and really work it into the mix. If your mix is really wet, it's probably already started foaming and the bath bomb mix is going to be no good. Your best bet at that point is to start over and make a new batch. You can dry out the mix and use it like you would bath salts if you don't want it to go to waste.

Toss a handful in the tub and you'll still get the oils, butters and salts you would from a bath bomb.

It's best to err on the side of making things too dry because it's easier to fix. Add ingredients and water or witch hazel slowly and keep a constant eye on the consistency as you mix things together. Don't be afraid to make adjustments on the fly. The ingredient lists in these recipes are nothing more than simple guidelines. There are outside factors like humidity that can affect the recipes and impact the quantity of wet and dry ingredients that need to be used.

Step 5: Pack the molds and then remove the bath bombs from the mold.

This is my favorite part. I pack the bath bomb molds as full of the bath bomb mix as I can get them and then really pack it in tight.

When using two-piece molds, I fill both halves to overflowing and then press the molds together while slowly twisting back and forth to really pack the mix into the molds. When using one-piece molds, I'll fill the one piece until it's overflowing and then flip it over and press it against a flat surface and slowly twist back and forth while pushing down until the mold is packed.

When done right, you'll be left with a single bath bomb that's ready to be removed from the mold and set out to dry. When done wrong, the bath bomb will break in half or crumble shortly after it comes out of the mold.

Be gentle when removing bath bombs from the molds because they're still wet and can crumble at the slightest touch. If you've got the consistency of the mix right, a gentle twisting motion should be all that's required to remove the bath bomb from the mold.

Step 6: Let the bath bombs dry and then use them or move them into storage.

Once you've removed the bath bombs from the molds, you're going to want to give them time to dry before attempting to handle them.

Leave them sitting in a cool, dry place for a day or two, until they feel hard to the touch. If all the stars aligned correctly, you'll be left with a bunch of bath bombs that can be used immediately or stored away in an airtight container for future use. Bath bombs will degrade quickly if they're exposed to heat or moisture, so it's important to keep them protected from light, air and moisture.

Use your bath bombs within a few months of making them for best results.

Chapter 5: Using Your Bath Bombs

You've done the hard part. Now comes the fun part—actually using the bath bombs.

Using bath bombs properly is very difficult, so pay close attention. Here are the steps required to use your bath bombs:

1. **Fill your tub with warm water.**
2. **Toss a bath bomb into the tub.**
3. **Climb in and enjoy the oils in the tub and the aromas that permeate the room.**

Now, for the hard part. You're eventually going to have to force yourself to get out of the tub, which can prove very difficult when you've got a great bath bomb going!

Chapter 6: The Basic Bath Bomb Recipes

Here's the basic bath bomb recipe that's used as the basis for most of the recipes in this book. Learn this one and you'll be able to make the rest of the recipes.

The Basic Bath Bomb Recipe

Gather the following:

- 2 cups baking soda.
- 1 cup citric acid.
- ¼ cup Epsom salt.
- ¼ cup corn starch.
- 2 tablespoons vegetable oil.
- A spray bottle with witch hazel.

Follow these directions:

1. Combine the baking soda, citric acid, Epsom salt and corn starch.
2. Slowly stir the vegetable oil into the dry ingredients. I recommend using coconut oil or sweet almond oil. If you use coconut oil and it's cold, you might have to melt the oil first.
3. Get the mix to the right consistency by lightly misting it with witch hazel and working it in.
4. Pack the bath bombs into the molds.
5. Remove the bath bombs from the molds.
6. Let the bath bombs dry overnight.

7. Store them in an airtight container in a cool, dry place.

Chapter 7: The No-Citric Acid Bomb

If you don't have access to citric acid, there's another ingredient you can use to make your bath bombs. Cream of tartar can be substituted for citric acid and will work for most bath bomb recipes. You won't get the rapid bubbling action that you do with citric acid, but it's an acceptable substitute.

When using cream of tartar as a replacement, you're going to want to cut the amount used down to half of what the recipe says is needed if you were to use citric acid. If you're making a recipe that calls for 2 cups of baking soda, all you're going to need as far as citric acid is concerned is half a cup.

Like the previous recipe, this is a basic recipe that you probably aren't going to want to use on its own. Add some essential oils in step 2 if you want to add fragrance and use this recipe as a jumping off point.

The No-Citric Acid Bomb Recipe

Gather the following:

- 2 cups baking soda.
- ½ cup cream of tartar.
- ¼ cup Epsom salt.
- ¼ cup corn starch.
- 2 tablespoons vegetable oil.
- A spray bottle with witch hazel.

Follow these directions:

1. Combine the baking soda, cream of tartar, Epsom salt and corn starch.
2. Slowly stir the vegetable oil into the dry ingredients. I recommend using coconut oil or sweet almond oil. If you use coconut oil and it's cold, you might have to melt the oil first.
3. Get the mix to the right consistency by lightly misting it with witch hazel and working it in.
4. Pack the bath bombs into the molds.
5. Remove the bath bombs from the molds.
6. Let the bath bombs dry overnight.
7. Store them in an airtight container in a cool, dry place.

Chapter 8: The Milk Bomb

We've been taught since we were little that *drinking* milk is good for our health, but relatively few people have been taught that milk can be applied *externally* to improve the health of our skin. The natural lactic acid found in milk helps exfoliate the skin, revealing the healthy skin trapped beneath all those dead skin cells.

The powdered milk added to this bath bomb recipe creates a rich, luxurious bath. We've also added cocoa butter to this recipe, which makes it even creamier. The fragrance is up to you. I've found citrus essential oils are a good match for this recipe. Try 5 to 10 drops of Bergamot oil to start.

The Milk Bomb Recipe

Gather the following:

- 2 cups baking soda.
- 1 cup citric acid.
- ¼ cup Epsom salt.
- ¼ cup powdered milk.
- 1 tablespoon coconut oil.
- 2 tablespoons cocoa butter.
- A spray bottle with witch hazel.

Follow these directions:

1. Combine the baking soda, citric acid, Epsom salt and powdered milk.

2. Melt the coconut oil and cocoa butter. Stir them together. If you're adding essential oils, let the melted butter/oil mixture cool a little before stirring them in.
3. Add the wet ingredients to the dry ingredients slowly and work them in.
4. Get the mix to the right consistency by lightly misting it with witch hazel and working it in.
5. Pack the bath bombs into the molds.
6. Remove the bath bombs from the molds.
7. Let the bath bombs dry overnight.
8. Store them in an airtight container in a cool, dry place.

Chapter 9: The Lavender Bomb

This is the first recipe in the book that calls for a specific essential oil. Lavender essential oil is the top-selling essential oil of all time because it can be used for all sorts of therapeutic reasons, and the risk associated with use of this oil is minimal. Most people who start using essential oils start with lavender oil and expand out from there.

Lavender oil has withstood the test of time and has been used for many years as an effective home remedy against acne, sunburns, burns and a number of other skin conditions. It's been shown to numb pain, it can help heal wounds and it has a relaxing fragrance. As is the case with all essential oils, there is the risk of skin irritation or an allergic reaction, but most people are able to use lavender oil safely.

The Lavender Bomb Recipe

Gather the following:

- 2 cups baking soda.
- 1 cup citric acid.
- ¼ cup Epsom salt.
- ¼ cup corn starch.
- 10 to 15 drops lavender essential oil.
- 2 tablespoons sweet almond oil.
- A spray bottle with witch hazel.

Follow these directions:

1. Combine the baking soda, citric acid, Epsom salt and corn starch.
2. Mix the sweet almond oil and the lavender essential oil. Slowly stir the oil mix into the dry ingredients.
3. Get the mix to the right consistency by lightly misting it with witch hazel and working it in.
4. Pack the bath bombs into the molds.
5. Remove the bath bombs from the molds.
6. Let the bath bombs dry overnight.
7. Store them in an airtight container in a cool, dry place.

Chapter 10: Flower Petal Bombs

These bath bombs take the basic bath bomb recipe and add flower petals to the dry ingredients. You can use rose petals, lavender petals, chamomile petals or the petals from a number of other flowers to create a luxurious bath experience where you feel like a beautiful princess floating in a tub infused with flowers.

Of course these recipes can get a little messy, so if you want a similar experience minus the clean-up at the end, you can toss your bath bomb into a nylon stocking before throwing it in the tub.

Flower petal bombs work best when scented with a floral oil that's similar to the type of petals that were used. Lavender petal bombs should be scented with lavender essential oil; rose petal bombs should be scented with rose oil, and so on. I've included a couple of flower petal bomb recipes in this chapter, but there's no reason to limit yourself to these recipes. Once you've made one flower petal bomb recipe, you can pretty much make them all.

The Basic Flower Bomb Recipe

Gather the following:

- 2 cups baking soda.
- 1 cup citric acid.
- ¼ cup Epsom salt.
- ¼ cup corn starch.
- Dried flower petals.
- 5 to 10 drops floral essential oil.

- 2 tablespoons sweet almond oil.
- A spray bottle with witch hazel.

Follow these directions:

1. Combine the baking soda, citric acid, Epsom salt and corn starch. Add the dried flower petals to the mix and stir them in.
2. Mix the sweet almond oil and the floral essential oil. Slowly stir the oil mix into the dry ingredients.
3. Get the mix to the right consistency by lightly misting it with witch hazel and working it in.
4. Pack the bath bombs into the molds. For aesthetic value, you can add several dried flower petals to the bottom of each mold before pressing the mix into the molds.
5. Remove the bath bombs from the molds.
6. Let the bath bombs dry overnight.
7. Store them in an airtight container in a cool, dry place.

The Rose Bomb Recipe

This recipe calls for rose petals and rose essential oil. Rose oil has an intoxicating fragrance that balances the mind and spirit while invigorating the body. It's a great oil to use when skin care is of utmost concern, and it's the perfect oil for dry and aging skin.

Be prepared for sticker shock if you decide to buy rose essential oil, since a small bottle of pure oil will set you back a couple hundred bucks. If you want a less expensive option, go with rose geranium oil or rose absolute.

Gather the following:

- 2 cups baking soda.
- 1 cup citric acid.
- ¼ cup Epsom salt.
- ¼ cup corn starch.
- Dried rose petals.
- 5 to 10 drops rose essential oil.
- 2 tablespoons sweet almond oil.
- A spray bottle with witch hazel.

Follow these directions:

1. Combine the baking soda, citric acid, Epsom salt and corn starch. Crumble the dried rose petals and stir them in.
2. Mix the sweet almond oil and the rose essential oil. Slowly stir the oil mix into the dry ingredients.
3. Get the mix to the right consistency by lightly misting it with witch hazel and working it in.
4. Pack the bath bombs into the molds. For aesthetic value, you can add several dried rose petals to the bottom of each mold before pressing the mix into the molds.
5. Remove the bath bombs from the molds.
6. Let the bath bombs dry overnight.

7. Store them in an airtight container in a cool, dry place.

The Lavender Petal Bomb Recipe

Gather the following:

- 2 cups baking soda.
- 1 cup citric acid.
- ¼ cup Epsom salt.
- ¼ cup corn starch.
- Dried lavender flowers.
- 5 to 10 drops lavender essential oil.
- 2 tablespoons sweet almond oil.
- A spray bottle with witch hazel.

Follow these directions:

1. Combine the baking soda, citric acid, Epsom salt and corn starch. Crumble the dried lavender flowers and stir them in.
2. Mix the sweet almond oil and the lavender essential oil. Slowly stir the oil mix into the dry ingredients.
3. Get the mix to the right consistency by lightly misting it with witch hazel and working it in.
4. Pack the bath bombs into the molds. For aesthetic value, you can add several lavender flowers to the bottom of each mold before pressing the mix into the molds.
5. Remove the bath bombs from the molds.
6. Let the bath bombs dry overnight.

7. Store them in an airtight container in a cool, dry place.

The German Chamomile Petal Bomb Recipe

If you haven't been around essential oils before, you may not have heard of German chamomile. It's a blue oil that has a light, grassy fragrance with hints of apple. It's soothing and relaxing and has antioxidant and anti-inflammatory properties.

German chamomile oil is said to help support healthy skin, so it's a good choice for bath bombs. Don't get German chamomile mixed up with Roman chamomile. While they share the chamomile moniker, the oils smell different and have slightly different properties. While Roman chamomile can be used in bath care products as well, it has a campherous fragrance that doesn't meld well with German chamomile.

Gather the following:

- 2 cups baking soda.
- 1 cup citric acid.
- ¼ cup Epsom salt.
- ¼ cup corn starch.
- Dried German chamomile flowers.
- 5 to 10 drops German chamomile essential oil.
- 2 tablespoons sweet almond oil.
- A spray bottle with witch hazel.

Follow these directions:

1. Combine the baking soda, citric acid, Epsom salt and corn starch. Crumble the dried German chamomile flowers and stir them in.
2. Mix the sweet almond oil and the German chamomile essential oil. Slowly stir the oil mix into the dry ingredients.
3. Get the mix to the right consistency by lightly misting it with witch hazel and working it in.
4. Pack the bath bombs into the molds. For aesthetic value, you can add several German chamomile flowers to the bottom of each mold before pressing the mix into the molds.
5. Remove the bath bombs from the molds.
6. Let the bath bombs dry overnight.
7. Store them in an airtight container in a cool, dry place.

Chapter 11: White Tea Bombs

White tea is believed to help slow the effects of aging and can be used to help rejuvenate dry, damaged skin. It has anti-inflammatory properties and may help protect the skin from damage from UV rays.

If you don't have white tea on hand, you might be able to get the same effect from green tea. Regardless of the type of tea used, you want to brew it much stronger than you would if you were planning on drinking the tea. I use 4 to 5 white tea bags and let them steep for 30 to 45 minutes.

Instead of water or witch hazel, I use white tea in the spray bottle for this recipe in order to get as much white tea into the recipe as possible.

This recipe isn't going to have much fragrance on its own. Feel free to add your favorite essential oils to the recipe to add fragrance.

White Tea Bombs Recipe

Gather the following:

- 2 cups baking soda.
- 1 cup citric acid.
- ¼ cup Epsom salt.
- ¼ cup corn starch.
- 2 tablespoons strong white tea.
- 2 tablespoons sweet almond oil.
- A spray bottle with strong white tea.

Follow these directions:

1. Combine the baking soda, citric acid, Epsom salt and corn starch.
2. Mix the sweet almond oil and strong white tea. Add any essential oils you plan on using at this time. Slowly stir the oil mix into the dry ingredients.
3. Get the mix to the right consistency by lightly misting it with white tea and working it in until it's the right consistency.
4. Pack the bath bombs into the molds.
5. Remove the bath bombs from the molds.
6. Let the bath bombs dry overnight.
7. Store them in an airtight container in a cool, dry place.

Chapter 12: Cinnamon Sugar Bombs

Cinnamon sugar bombs add cinnamon and sugar to the mix to create a bath bomb that will leave you smelling great. The cinnamon plumps the skin up a bit and can help eliminate fine lines and small wrinkles. It cleanses the skin and has seen use as a home remedy for eczema and acne. Cinnamon is also thought to help reduce the effects of aging. This recipe calls for cinnamon tea as the method of adding cinnamon to the recipe.

The sugar is added to this recipe in the form of raw honey because it has antibacterial and antimicrobial properties. Honey soothes the skin and contains natural antioxidants.

Cinnamon Sugar Bomb Recipe

Gather the following:

- 2 cups baking soda.
- 1 cup citric acid.
- ¼ cup Epsom salt.
- ¼ cup corn starch.
- 2 tablespoons cinnamon tea.
- 1 tablespoon raw honey.
- 2 tablespoons coconut oil.
- A spray bottle with cinnamon tea.

Follow these directions:

1. Combine the baking soda, citric acid, Epsom salt and corn starch.
2. Melt the coconut oil. Add the cinnamon tea and raw honey to the coconut oil and whisk them together. Slowly stir the oil mix into the dry ingredients.
3. Get the mix to the right consistency by lightly misting it with cinnamon tea and working it in.
4. Pack the bath bombs into the molds.
5. Remove the bath bombs from the molds.
6. Let the bath bombs dry overnight.
7. Store them in an airtight container in a cool, dry place.

Chapter 13: Peppermint Sage Bombs

This bath bomb adds a couple new essential oils to the mix that we haven't used yet. Peppermint essential oil is a powerful essential oil that has a strong mint fragrance. It's beneficial to the respiratory system and may help with congestion and coughing. It's also a good skin care oil that has a cooling effect when applied topically.

Sage essential oil is strongly antifungal and antimicrobial and can help the body fight off internal and external infections. It can be used to help eliminate scars and will speed up the healing process when applied to damaged skin.

Peppermint Sage Bombs Recipe

Gather the following:

- 2 cups baking soda.
- 1 cup citric acid.
- ¼ cup Epsom salt.
- ¼ cup corn starch.
- 2 tablespoons coconut oil.
- 5 drops peppermint essential oil.
- 10 drops sage essential oil.
- A spray bottle with witch hazel.

Follow these directions:

1. Combine the baking soda, citric acid, Epsom salt and corn starch.

2. Melt the coconut oil and let it cool for a few minutes. Add the essential oils to the coconut oil and whisk them together. Slowly stir the oil mix into the dry ingredients.
3. Get the mix to the right consistency by lightly misting it with witch hazel and working it in.
4. Pack the bath bombs into the molds.
5. Remove the bath bombs from the molds.
6. Let the bath bombs dry overnight.
7. Store them in an airtight container in a cool, dry place.

Chapter 14: Citrus Bombs

There are a number of different citrus essential oils that can be used to create this recipe. I've tried grapefruit, Bergamot, lemon and lime, and they've all worked well. Citrus oils are cleansing by nature, and they'll leave you feeling happy and invigorated. When I'm feeling down in the dumps, I use a citrus bomb, and it usually gets me feeling better in no time at all.

This recipe adds Shea butter to the mix. This butter has healing properties and is a great oil to use to moisturize dry skin. If you've got redness or inflammation you want to get rid of, Shea butter is a good option.

Citrus Bombs Recipe

Gather the following:

- 2 cups baking soda.
- 1 cup citric acid.
- ¼ cup Epsom salt.
- ¼ cup corn starch.
- 1 tablespoon Shea butter.
- 5 to 10 drops citrus essential oil.
- A spray bottle with witch hazel.

Follow these directions:

1. Combine the baking soda, citric acid, Epsom salt and corn starch.

2. Melt the Shea butter and let it cool for a few minutes. Add the essential oil to the butter and whisk them together. Slowly stir the mixture into the dry ingredients.
3. Get the mix to the right consistency by lightly misting it with witch hazel and working it in.
4. Pack the bath bombs into the molds.
5. Remove the bath bombs from the molds.
6. Let the bath bombs dry overnight.
7. Store them in an airtight container in a cool, dry place.

Chapter 14: Moisturizing Bomb

Take Aloe vera butter and sweet almond oil and combine it with sandalwood essential oil and what do you get? A bath bomb that smells great and has strong moisturizing properties. Use this bath bomb when you've got dry skin and it'll soon be a thing of the past.

Moisturizing Bomb Recipe

Gather the following:

- 2 cups baking soda.
- 1 cup citric acid.
- ¼ cup Epsom salt.
- ¼ cup corn starch.
- 1 tablespoon sweet almond oil.
- 2 tablespoons Aloe vera butter.
- 10 drops sandalwood essential oil.
- A spray bottle with witch hazel.

Follow these directions:

1. Combine the baking soda, citric acid, Epsom salt and corn starch.
2. Melt the Aloe vera butter and let it cool for a few minutes. Add the sweet almond oil and the essential oils and whisk them together. Slowly stir the oil mix into the dry ingredients.
3. Get the mix to the right consistency by lightly misting it with witch hazel and working it in.

4. Pack the bath bombs into the molds.
5. Remove the bath bombs from the molds.
6. Let the bath bombs dry overnight.
7. Store them in an airtight container in a cool, dry place.

Chapter 15: Christmas Anytime Bomb

One of my favorite fragrances is the smell of a fresh-cut Christmas tree sitting in my living room. Christmas is one of my favorite times of year, and smelling the fragrance of pine essential oils evokes feelings of Christmas joy in me.

Pine essential oil can be used as a home remedy for a number of skin conditions, including rashes, eczema, scabies, cuts, burns and infections. It renews the skin while balancing sebum production. It also has analgesic properties, so a soak in the tub with a pine oil bath bomb may help relieve aches and pains.

Christmas Anytime Bomb Recipe

Gather the following:

- 2 cups baking soda.
- 1 cup citric acid.
- ¼ cup Epsom salt.
- ¼ cup corn starch.
- 2 tablespoons sweet almond oil.
- 5 to 10 drops pine essential oil.
- A spray bottle with witch hazel.

Follow these directions:

1. Combine the baking soda, citric acid, Epsom salt and corn starch.

2. Add the pine essential oil to the sweet almond oil and whisk them together. Slowly stir the oil mix into the dry ingredients.
3. Get the mix to the right consistency by lightly misting it with witch hazel and working it in.
4. Pack the bath bombs into the molds.
5. Remove the bath bombs from the molds.
6. Let the bath bombs dry overnight.
7. Store them in an airtight container in a cool, dry place.

Chapter 16: Tequila Lime Bombs

Here's a festive bath bomb that combines tequila and lime essential oil to create a soothing bath experience that works well to help heal damaged skin. Just be careful not to drink too much of the tequila while making these bombs or you might end up with skin that's in worse shape instead of better!

Tequila Lime Bombs Recipe

Gather the following:

- 2 cups baking soda.
- 1 cup citric acid.
- ¼ cup Epsom salt.
- ¼ cup corn starch.
- 1 tablespoon lime zest.
- 2 tablespoons coconut oil.
- 5 to 10 drops lime essential oil.
- A spray bottle with agave tequila.

Follow these directions:

1. Combine the baking soda, citric acid, Epsom salt, lime zest and corn starch.
2. Melt the coconut oil and let it cool for a few minutes. Add the lime essential oil to the coconut oil and whisk them together. Slowly stir the oil mix into the dry ingredients.

3. Get the mix to the right consistency by lightly misting it with tequila and working it in.
4. Pack the bath bombs into the molds.
5. Remove the bath bombs from the molds.
6. Let the bath bombs dry overnight.
7. Store them in an airtight container in a cool, dry place.

Chapter 17: Triple Lemon Bomb

The triple lemon bomb calls for three different lemon ingredients to create a bath bomb that smells lemon fresh and features a number of benefits. Lemon butter is a lesser-known ingredient that's made from oils and waxes that are taken from lemon peels. It contains compounds that are anti-inflammatory and will help protect the skin. It also has moisturizing and skin toning properties.

Lemon essential oil also has toning properties and may be helpful in removing cellulite. The fragrance of lemon essential oil can help you focus and will allow you to think clearly.

Triple Lemon Bomb Recipe

Gather the following:

- 2 cups baking soda.
- 1 cup citric acid.
- ¼ cup Epsom salt.
- ¼ cup corn starch.
- 1 tablespoon lemon zest.
- 2 tablespoons lemon butter.
- 5 drops lemon essential oil.
- A spray bottle with witch hazel.

Follow these directions:

1. Combine the baking soda, citric acid, Epsom salt, lemon zest and corn starch.

2. Melt the lemon butter and let it cool for a few minutes. Add the lemon essential oil to the melted butter and whisk them together. Slowly stir the oil mix into the dry ingredients.
3. Get the mix to the right consistency by lightly misting it with witch hazel and working it in.
4. Pack the bath bombs into the molds.
5. Remove the bath bombs from the molds.
6. Let the bath bombs dry overnight.
7. Store them in an airtight container in a cool, dry place.

Chapter 18: Bath Bomb Wands

This recipe can be made using any of the previous recipes in the book. All you have to do is replace the corn starch with kaolin clay, which hardens up to keep the bath bombs on the wands. You're going to need some thin 8- to 12-inch wooden dowels to make your bath bomb wands with.

Peppermint Sage Bombs Recipe

Gather the following:

- 2 cups baking soda.
- 1 cup citric acid.
- ¼ cup Epsom salts.
- ¼ cup kaolin clay.
- 2 tablespoons coconut oil.
- 5 to 10 drops of your favorite essential oil.
- A spray bottle with witch hazel.

Follow these directions:

1. Combine the baking soda, citric acid, Epsom salt and kaolin clay.
2. Melt the coconut oil and let it cool for a few minutes. Add the essential oil to the coconut oil and whisk them together. Slowly stir the oil mix into the dry ingredients.
3. Get the mix to the right consistency by lightly misting it with witch hazel and working it in.

4. Pack the bath bombs into the molds.
5. Slowly press a wooden dowel into the center of the bath bomb.
6. Remove the bath bombs from the molds.
7. Let the bath bombs dry overnight.
8. Store them in an airtight container in a cool, dry place.
9. When you want to use these bath bombs, you can hold them by the stick and swish them back and forth in the tub, leaving a trail of bubbles behind the wand as it moves.

Chapter 19: Shower Bombs

If you don't have a bathtub (or you just don't like baths), don't worry. You can still enjoy great fragrances while you get clean. Shower bombs are like bath bombs, but they're made with kaolin clay so that they last a long time in the shower, releasing great fragrances the entire time.

This shower bomb calls for eucalyptus essential oil, but you could just as easily substitute other essential oils into the recipe. Use this bath bomb when you've got a cold or allergies have you feeling all congested and stuffed up. Breathe deeply and you might be able to clear up some of the congestion.

Shower bombs use more essential oils than bath bombs and should not be used in the bath.

Shower Bombs Recipe

Gather the following:

- 2 cups baking soda.
- 1 cup citric acid.
- ¼ cup Epsom salts.
- ¼ cup kaolin clay.
- 2 tablespoons cocoa butter.
- 20 to 30 drops of your favorite essential oil.
- A spray bottle with witch hazel.

Follow these directions:

1. Combine the baking soda, citric acid, Epsom salt, kaolin clay and corn starch.
2. Melt the cocoa oil and let it cool for a few minutes. Add the essential oils to the coconut oil and whisk them together. Slowly stir the oil mix into the dry ingredients.
3. Get the mix to the right consistency by lightly misting it with witch hazel and working it in.
4. Pack the shower bombs into the molds.
5. Remove the shower bombs from the molds.
6. Let the shower bombs dry overnight.
7. Store them in an airtight container in a cool, dry place.
8. When you want to use these shower bombs, all you have to do is turn on the shower and place one on the floor where it'll come in contact with the stream of water.

FAQ – Frequently Asked Questions

I've compiled answers to some of the more common questions people have when they start making bath bombs. If a question or problem comes up, check here first to see if the question has been answered.

What will the mixture feel like when it's damp enough?

This is a tough one to explain in writing. I've heard it compared to damp sand, which is close, but isn't exactly dead-on. The best way to check your mix is to squeeze it and make sure it retains its shape.

Does the mixing have to be done by hand?

No, you can use an electric stand mixer to thoroughly mix the ingredients if you'd like. Place the ingredients into the mixer, set it to low and let it run until the ingredients are combined.

This can get a little messy due to the powdered ingredients. To prevent the powder from getting everywhere, place a towel over the electric mixer while it's doing its thing.

Why won't my bath bombs stick together?

The most common reason for this is too much oil was used. Reduce the amount of oil used in future recipes to see if this solves the problem.

Can I use other essential oils?

It depends on the essential oil. Make sure any other oils you use are safe for contact with the skin and that you're able to tolerate them. You don't want to have an allergic reaction after coating your whole body with essential oils as you climb in and out of the tub.

There are some essential oils that aren't safe for use, so it's important you do your due diligence. You should also check with your physician before starting to use a new oil.

Why did my bath bombs crack and crumble?

This can happen for a number of reasons. Here are some of the more common reasons this happens:

- Too much of one of the dry ingredients was used.
- There wasn't enough witch hazel or water added.
- The mixture was allowed to sit for too long before it was packed into the mold.
- The bath bombs weren't carefully removed from the mold.
- The bath bomb wasn't packed tightly enough.

Why did my bath bombs expand out of the mold?

This can happen when there's too much moisture in the bath bomb mix. It's also a common occurrence when bath bombs are made during days with high humidity.

Why is the bath bomb mix fizzing?

You added too much liquid and it set off the citric acid and baking soda. If it's a small reaction, you might be able to stir things up and get it to stop. If it's a big reaction, you're probably going to have to start over.

How Do I Add Color to the Bath Bombs?

There are a number of ways bath bombs can be colored. Here are some of the more common methods:

- **Food coloring or food dyes.**
- **Natural clays.**
- **Bath bomb dyes.**
- **Soap colorants.**
- **Organic dyes.**

When choosing a color to use in your bath bombs, make sure that it's safe for contact with your skin, and that it won't stain your skin or your tub. You don't want to get out of the tub and find that your skin and your tub has been dyed that awesome neon purple color you found online.